# EKG and ECG Interpretation

## Learn EKG Interpretation, Rhythms, and Arrhythmia Fast!

# Table of Contents

# Introduction

I want to thank you and congratulate you for downloading the book, "EKG and ECG Interpretation".

This book contains helpful information about ECG interpretation, and how to interpret a range of different heartbeats and rhythms.

You will discover exactly what ECG interpretation is, how it is conducted, and the equipment required. You will learn about the different types of ECG, and how each one is performed and recorded.

You'll be shown how to read an ECG graph, and determine if a heartbeat is regular or not. This includes determining different ailments, heart rate, rhythm, and looking out for arrhythmias.

This book will provide you the steps and strategies required to successfully understand and interpret the different heart rhythms, and determine if your heart is functioning properly!

Thanks again for downloading this book, I hope you enjoy it!

# Chapter 1:
# The Basics of EKG/ECG

Electrocardiogram (ECG) is a combination of three words – electro, cardio, and gram, which mean electricity, heart, and recording, respectively. Simply put, it is a recording of the electrical activity of the heart. ECG is a non-invasive diagnostic procedure that can help determine the condition of the heart to a certain degree. It is also known as EKG because of the Greek word "kardia" for heart.

## Review of the Cardiovascular System

To understand ECG better and the steps in interpreting it, a review of the anatomy and physiology of the heart is important. Here it is:

The heart is a muscular organ made up of four chambers, two atria (right and left) and two ventricles (right and left). Its size is estimated to be that of the size of a person's closed fist. It acts as the pump to circulate oxygenated blood from the heart to the vital organs first, then to the remaining parts of the body. Together with the lungs and vascular system, the heart works to turn deoxygenated (oxygen deprived) blood to oxygenated blood for distribution around the body.

## Blood Flow through the Heart

It is also important to know how blood flows through the heart into all body parts. Starting on the heart's right upper chamber called the right atrium, the deoxygenated blood from the upper extremities and head will enter the heart via the superior vena cava. The blood coming from the lower parts of the body would enter the right atrium through the inferior vena cava. Oxygen deprived blood from the heart itself will go back to the heart via the coronary sinus.

From the right atrium, blood would pass through the tricuspid valve going to the right ventricle. The tricuspid prevents the backflow of blood from ventricle to atrium, as blood flow is unidirectional or flows in one direction only. From the right ventricle, blood will pass through the pulmonary artery, which is the only artery that carries deoxygenated blood. It would go to the lungs where gas exchange takes place. In here, the release of carbon dioxide and the absorption of oxygen will take place, making the deoxygenated blood become oxygenated blood.

The oxygenated blood will go back to the heart through the pulmonary vein, which is the only vein that carries oxygenated blood, to the left atrium. Then it will pass through the bicuspid valve to go to the left ventricle. Just like the tricuspid valve, the bicuspid valve will prevent the backflow of the blood. From the left ventricle, it would pass through the semilunar aortic valve, aorta and then to the systemic circulation. This cycle would then be repeated.

Your heart pumps around 5-6 liters of blood per minute, totaling to 7200-7500 liters throughout a whole day. The normal average heartbeat for adults is about 80-100 per minute.

With this knowledge, it will be easier to understand the conduction system or the electrical activity of the heart, which is the main purpose of ECG.

## Understanding the Conduction System

The conduction system is why your heart pumps. How does this happen? Just like a regular pump machine that needs a power source and electricity for it to run, the heart needs electricity, too. The difference is that the heart is able to create the electrical impulses that it needs and controls the impulses through a specialized conduction pathway.

This conduction pathway is composed of the following:

> ➤ The Sino-atrial node or SA node

> ➤ The Atrio-ventricular node or AV node

> ➤ The bundle of His

> ➤ The left and right bundle

> ➤ The Purkinje fibers

The SA node is known as the pacemaker of the heart as it is the one that initiates the impulse. From the SA node, the electric impulse will travel up to the AV node. From the AV node, the impulse will pass to the bundle of His. It will continue downward to the left and right bundles. Finally, the last destination of the impulse is at the Purkinje fibers. This is equivalent to one rhythmic heartbeat.

In a normal person, this will occur 80-100 times per minute. In case the SA node fails to transmit an impulse, the AV node will take over. However, it can only do as many as 40 to 60 impulses, giving 40-60 beats per minute (bpm). Again, if the AV node fails, the survival instinct of the body will take over and the bundle of His will take over. It can generate up to 20 to 40 impulses only. Still, if that fails, the Purkinje fiber will take the role of the SA node, but its capacity is only 0-20 impulses.

## *The purpose of ECG*

This is where ECG comes in. As the impulses will initiate the rhythmic beat of the heart, any deviation from what this system normally does can affect the whole body. Hence, it is very important to assess the condition of the conduction system, especially to those with existing cardiovascular disorders.

# Chapter 2:
# Electrocardiogram: Uses, Procedure and Types

ECG or EKG is a painless diagnostic exam that is helpful in determining any abnormality of the structure, function and rhythm of the heart.

## *Uses of ECG*

The doctor may order ECG to determine the following:

➢ The condition of the conduction system or electrical activity of the heart

➢ The rate of the heart

➢ The rhythm of the heart

➢ The presence of ischemia (poor blood flow)

➢ The occurrence of a heart attack

➢ The cause of a chest pain

➢ Hypertrophy or enlargement of the chambers of the heart

➢ Other structural deviations such as obstructions, holes, thickening of lining or stenosis (narrowing) of valves, to name a few

Aside from these, the doctor may also order ECG for the following reasons:

➢ For complaints of shortness of breath, fainting, dizziness or palpitations

> To determine if the cardiac medicines prescribed to a person are working

> If a device, such as a pacemaker implant, is functioning well

> To monitor the health of the heart of those with a family history of cardiac ailments and other medical conditions such as hypertension, diabetes, coronary artery disorders, atherosclerosis, kidney problems and others

## Step-by-Step Procedure of ECG

The electrocardiogram procedure can be performed in the clinic of the doctor or in the patient's hospital room (if he or she is confined). There is no special preparation required for this exam.

Here are the needed materials:

> ECG machine

> ECG paper or strip

> 10 sticky pads to attach the electrodes

> Wipes

> Razor (for hairy chest)

## Before the Test

1. One should not take any medicine that may affect the results of ECG. Examples are cardiac and antidepressant drugs.

2.  Preferably, the patient will have not taken any stimulants such as coffee, tea or sodas as these products can alter the rate and rhythm of the heart.

3.  The patient should rest well prior to the test. He or she should not have done a strenuous or heavy workout prior to the exam.

## How to do the Test?

Here are the steps to take to do a standard (also known as routine or resting) ECG.

1.  The technician would explain the procedure to the patient and its importance. They should wash and sanitize their hands.

2.  They should also provide privacy through proper screening of the bed or room, as the patient will have to remove their top or shirt. Having a chaperone is allowed.

3.  Patient assumes a supine or lying position. In case the patient cannot tolerate this position, ECG procedure can be done in a semi-Fowler's position or in a more upright position.

4.  In the case of the patient having a hairy chest, it is sometimes necessary to shave off some of the hair because it may interfere with the results of the test. The chest must also be dry.

5.  Electrodes will be attached to the patient. There is a standardized system for the placement of the ten electrodes – four electrodes on the extremities and six

on the chest wall. This will produce the 12 electrical views of the patient's heart.

a.  Right wrist or shoulder

b.  Left wrist or shoulder

c.  Right ankle

d.  Left ankle

e.  V1 - 4<sup>th</sup> intercostal space on the right sternal edge

f.  V2 – 4<sup>th</sup> intercostal space on the left sternal edge

g.  V3 – midway between v2 and V4

h.  V4 –5<sup>th</sup> intercostal space at mid-clavicular line

i.  V5 - 5<sup>th</sup> intercostal space (same level as V4) but on anterior axillary line

j.  V6 – on the same level as V4 and V5 but on horizontal mid-axillary line.

The leads are color-coded: red, green, black and white. The AHA (American heart Institute) follows this code for the extremities:

k.  Red (left leg)

l.  Green (right leg)

m. Black (left arm)

n.  White (right arm)

For the chest wall, this is the color code:

a. V1 – brown/red

b. V2 – brown/yellow

c. V3 – brown/green

d. V4 – brown/blue

e. V5 – brown/orange

f. V6 – brown/purple

Do not worry if you feel that you wouldn't be able to memorize this color-coding. Most of the time, there is an indicated guide to where the placement of electrodes should be on the lead itself.

Place the electrodes carefully because incorrect placement will most likely produce inaccurate results.

6. The patient should be very still while the machine is running. Any movement can interfere with the results of the test. The electrical activity of the heart will be recorded and translated on paper.

7. After the exam, remove the electrodes and wipe off the sticky pads with the wipes.

*Tests may have incorrect results due to the following:*

➢ The electrodes are not securely attached to the skin.

➢ The patient was not still during the test.

> ➤ The patient took medicines or did a strenuous workout prior to the exam.

> ➤ The patient was stressed or heavily breathing.

## _Different Types of ECG/EKG_

Unknown to many people, there are several types of ECG or EKG aside from the routine ECG discussed above. Here are four of them.

1. Stress or Exercise ECG. This test takes 15 to 30 minutes. Just like in the standard ECG, electrodes will be placed on your chest wall. However, instead of lying down, this type determines the electrical activity of the heart while you are up and active.

   You would be asked to either walk or run a treadmill, or to cycle a stationary bike. If one cannot do it (for example because of a physical disability) then the technician will induce a similar effect of exercise or activity through medicines.

   At the beginning, your exercise is light and at a slow pace. Later on though, the technician will increase the speed and add a slope to make it harder for you. This will cause your heart to work harder, too. From there, the technician and the doctor will be able to monitor the function of your heart during stress or hard work.

   You can ask the technician or doctor to stop the test at any time, especially if you are feeling unwell or having chest pain. As your doctor will need to monitor your blood pressure and heart rate along with ECG, they may stop the test if your BP or heart rate suddenly increases or you experience shortness of breath.

2. 24-Hour ECG or Holter monitoring. This is also known as Continuous ECG. In this test, electrodes will be placed on your chest wall. These electrodes are connected to a portable tape recorder. The recorder, on the other hand, is attached to a belt. You need to wear this device for 24 hours doing your daily regular routine. You would be asked to record all your activities including this information: time, activity that you are doing and the symptoms that you feel. It is not advisable to take a shower or bath during the time you are wearing the device. After the 24 hours, you can remove the device and return it to the doctor for analysis.

3. Event recorder. This is similar to Holter monitoring or a 24-hour ECG. A device will also be attached to the patient. However, you would only record in the diary the symptoms and time of their occurrences. Then you can send the ECG readings to your doctor as soon as possible.

4. Implantable Loop Recorder (ILR). This single-lead ECG device is implanted in the left parasternal region of the chest. This is especially useful in monitoring the electrical activity of the patient's heart with recurrent but unexplainable episodes of palpitations, or for patients with atrial fibrillation or with genetic cardiac disorders.

# Chapter 3:
# Electrocardiogram: Basic Analysis and Interpretation of Rhythm and Rate

The skill of analyzing and interpreting the ECG results takes practice. First, you need to take a look at the features of the ECG paper and learn the different waveforms before you can start interpreting the results.

## ECG Paper

The results of the ECG will be recorded on an ECG paper or strip. This is a grid paper. The paper is divided into small and large squares or boxes. The lines of the large squares are dark. Each large square is five small squares high and five small squares long, totaling to 25 small squares per big square.

One small square is equivalent to 0.04 seconds. Since a big square is made up of five small squares, one big square is equivalent to .20 seconds. Therefore, five big boxes are equivalent to one second. The horizontal axis of the paper is about time. On top of the paper, you will see black marks at 3-second intervals.

The vertical axis, on the other hand, is about voltage or amplitude. On the vertical axis, two large squares or boxes are equivalent to 1 millivolt or mV while one small box is 0.1 mV.

## Waves of ECG

Electrical events during the ECG test will be translated onto the ECG paper into waveform components. It is necessary to recognize the different waves in the ECG paper. The following descriptions of waves are with respect to Lead II. Here they are:

P wave - This is the first deflection. It should be in the positive deflection. This represents atrial depolarization or the contraction of the atrium.

QRS complex - Starts with a negative deflection, the Q wave. It is then followed by an upward deflection, the R and finally a downward deflection again, the S. This represents ventricular depolarization or contraction of the ventricles.

T wave - It is a positive deflection. T waves represent ventricular repolarization or resting of the ventricles.

U wave - Sometimes, this does not appear in the trace and there is no reason for alarm. This represents the recovery of the Purkinje fibers.

Basing from these waves, you would be able to recognize other nomenclatures such as the following:

PR Interval – This is the period starting from atrial contraction up to ventricular contraction.

QT interval – This represents the start of ventricular contraction until its rest.

ST segment – This starts from the ending of ventricular contraction until its rest.

## Interpreting the Results

You can check eight things using the results of the ECG test. Again, this is in referral to Lead II results. Here they are:

- Rhythm

- Rate

- P Wave

- PR Interval

- QRS Interval

- T Wave

- QT Interval

- ST Segment

In this Chapter, interpretation of rhythm and rate will be discussed, while the next six items will be covered in the next chapter.

## Check the Rhythm

There are two ways to do this.

I. The paper and pencil method.

1. Examine the R to R intervals. On the paper, place a mark where the first R is, and then the second R. Then using the marked paper, check all the R-R intervals on the strip. Here are the things you should look for:

    a. Is there an equal space between all the R-R intervals? A 10% variation in the intervals is considered as normal.

    b. Is the rhythm regular? Or is there an increasing R-R duration?

    c. You can also check for atrial rhythm by measuring the P to P intervals instead. Again, observe the pattern closely.

II. Use of caliper method.

1. Set the caliper on the first and second R on the strip. When the caliper is set, measure the rest of the R-R intervals and check for regularity or consistency. If you notice that the set caliper is not the same for the other intervals, then that means that the rhythm is not regular. The questions and activities for a-c of the paper and pencil method also apply in this method.

## Check the Rate

There are several ways to do this:

First, count how many QRS complexes there are over a 6-second interval. Multiply the results by 10 and that is the heart rate. For example, if there are six QRS complexes in the 6-second interval, then the heart rate is 60. This method is useful both for regular and irregular rhythms.

The second method involves counting the number of small boxes within one R-R interval. Divide the number by 1500 and that is the heart rate. For example, if there are 22 small boxes in one R-R interval. The heart rate is 68 beats per minute (round off to the nearest 10).

Another method is dividing 300 over the number of large squares within one R-R interval. For example, if there are four large squares from one R to the next, then the heart rate is 75.

## Different Heart Rates

For adults:

- Normal HR is 60-100 beats/min

- Tachycardia (fast) more than 100 beats/min

- Bradycardia (slow) less than 60 beats/min

For children:

- Newborn to 12 months old– 100-160 beats/min

- 1- 2 years old – 90-150 beats/min

- 2-5 years old – 80-140 beats/min

- 6-12 years old – 70-120 beats/min

- more than 12 years old is the same as adults – 60-100 beats/min

# Chapter 4:
# ECG Interpretation for Waves and Intervals

In Chapter 3, you learned to analyze and interpret the rhythm and rate from an ECG test. In this chapter, you'll discover the methods used to analyze these six waves and intervals of the ECG test.

- P Wave

- PR Interval

- QRS Interval

- T Wave

- QT Interval

- ST Segment

## *Normal P Wave*

By plain observation and the counting of boxes, you can determine if the P wave is normal. When the atrium contracts or depolarizes, the normal amplitude is at 0.05 to 0.25 mV. This is equivalent to 0.5 to 2.5 small boxes on your ECG paper (vertical axis). For the duration, the normal is 0.06 to 0.11 seconds or 1.5 to 2.75 small boxes on the horizontal axis. The shape is smooth and rounded. It should also precede the QRS complex in a positive deflection.

When you look at the ECG strip, here are the things you need to answer concerning the P Wave.

1. Are they present? If the P wave is absent, it could mean that the atrium is not contracting properly or at all. There could be atrial fibrillation or sinus arrest.

2. Is the occurrence of the P waves regular? Intermittent appearance is also not a good sign of atrial depolarization.

3. For every QRS complex, is there a P wave that precedes it?

4. How does the P Wave look like? Are they smooth, rounded and in an upright position? Do they all look the same?

## *Normal PR Interval*

The PR interval measures the conduction time of AV (atrioventricular). You can measure the PR interval (from the P wave until the R wave of the QRS complex) using the following methods: paper and pencil, use of calipers, and the counting of small boxes or squares. The normal value is 0.12 to 0.20 seconds or equivalent to 3-5 small boxes in typical adults. It tends to be longer among the elderly. As the heart rate increases, the interval decreases.

Questions to ask:

1. Does the length of the PR Interval measure 3-5 small boxes or at 0.12 to 0.20 seconds?

2. In the whole Lead II, is the PR interval constant or varying?

## Normal QRS Interval

As the QRS complex determines ventricular contraction or depolarization, intervals of QRS complexes would therefore show the pattern of the contractions. The normal value is at 0.06 to 0.12 seconds or 1.5 to 3 small squares.

You measure the QRS interval from the ending of the PR interval until the end of the S wave. As with the PR interval, you can also use the three methods in determining the QRS interval. Look for the following:

1. Whether the range is within the normal values

2. Are the intervals regular or irregular?

3. What is the morphology of the QRS complex? If the complex is narrow, that could mean problems originating in the atrium, sinus, or in junction. If the complex is wide, then it could be of ventricular origin or possibly supraventricular with aberrant conduction.

## Normal T Wave

The T wave is a very good way to assess if the ventricles of the heart rest. After the QRS complex, there is a slight pause, followed by the T wave in a positive deflection. It is an asymmetrical waveform.

Watch out for the following abnormalities in T Waves:

- Inverted T waves – normal in children but indicative of many medical disorders in adults such as MI (myocardial infarction) Bundle branch block, and pulmonary embolism, just to name a few.

- Camel hump T waves – could be caused by hypokalemia (decreased potassium electrolytes) or tachycardia.

- Hyper acute T waves – seen in ST elevation-MI.

- Biphasic T waves – usually caused by Hypokalemia and myocardial ischemia.

- Flattened T waves – may represent hypokalemia and ischemia.

- In addition, T waves that are tall and very narrow with symmetrical peaks could be indicative of hyperkalemia or excessive potassium electrolytes in the blood.

## *Normal QT Interval*

Measure this from the beginning of the Q wave until the end of the T wave. Simply put, this is the period where the ventricle begins to contract until it rests. The normal value is at 0.36 to 0.44 seconds, or around 9-11 small squares. Of course, this could vary according to gender, age and heart rate of the patient.

If the QT interval is abnormally prolonged, it could be associated with ventricular arrhythmias. On the other hand, a congenital short QT interval syndrome is linked to the risk of atrial and ventricular fibrillation, and even sudden cardiac death.

## *Normal ST Segment*

The ST segment is the flat line that starts from the end of the QRS complex (ventricular contraction) until the beginning of the T wave (ventricular rest). It represents the early part of resting for the ventricle. This is also a very important detail to note as elevation or depression of this line is usually caused by myocardial ischemia or infarction.

## *Final Words on ECG Interpretation*

When you know the parts of the ECG paper and the nomenclatures plus the normal values, interpreting the ECG becomes very easy. Try to practice as much as you can with normal ECG results. When abnormal results occur, you will easily recognize where the deviation is and what could be the indication of that.

In the next chapter, you will learn about the different arrhythmias and their ECG results.

# Chapter 5:
# Irregular ECG Readings: Arrhythmias

Arrhythmia comes from the compound words "a", meaning without and "rhythmia", meaning rhythm. It is also called dysrhythmia. Many factors can cause arrhythmias such as:

➤ Problems in the structure and functions of the heart

➤ Presence of other medical conditions

➤ Smoking

➤ Too much alcohol or caffeine in the body

➤ Stress

There are different types of arrhythmias. It is possible to recognize each type based on the results of the ECG test. Here are some of them:

## *Atrial Tachycardia*

1. Atrial Fibrillation. The heart rate becomes rapid due to the chaotic weak atrial contractions. Although some atrial fibrillations are temporary, most episodes tend to worsen without proper treatment. If left untreated, this could lead to serious complications such as strokes.

   ECG Reading: There are no P waves, R-R intervals are irregular and the size of QRS complexes varies.

2. Atrial Flutter. Although it looks a lot like atrial fibrillation, there is more organization on rate and rhythm of the heart in atrial flutter. Still, just like atrial fibrillation, this too can lead to stroke.

ECG Reading: There are no P waves. There is a "Saw Tooth" pattern with a ratio of 2:1 or 3:1 with the QRS complexes. The PR Interval is not measurable.

3. Supraventricular Tachycardia. Supra means above so these forms of arrhythmias originate above the ventricles like in the atria or AV node. One example of this is Wolff-Parkinson-White Syndrome.

   ECG Reading: The P waves may look abnormal while the ventricular rhythm is regular.

## *Tachycardia in the Ventricles*

1. Ventricular Tachycardia (V-tach). This is a medical emergency characterized by a rapid heart rate with no sufficient delivery of blood to the vital organs and other body parts.

   ECG Reading: Highly recognizable. There are no P-waves, PR intervals are not measurable and the QRS complexes are wide and bizarre in appearance.

2. Ventricular Fibrillation. This emergency could be fatal if not managed within minutes. There are rapid, chaotic impulses from the ventricles, causing failures in delivering oxygenated blood to the vital organs.

   ECG Reading: ECG tracing looks like a wavy line. There are no P waves and QRS complexes. The rhythm is highly irregular.

## Bradycardia Arrhythmia

1.  Conduction block. This is when there is a delay or blockage of the impulses along the conduction pathway. It could be in the atria, ventricles or bundle of His. An example is if the conduction block is in the bundle of His, the delayed impulse is to the left and right side of your heart.

    In the ECG Reading, the rhythm is regular and the P wave and PR interval are both normal. The QRS is wider than normal.

## Premature Heart Beat

1.  Premature Ventricular Contractions (PVC). This is the most common arrhythmia and it can occur even to people who do not have heart ailments. In layman's term, this is when your heart skips a beat. It could be due to stress and too much exercise, caffeine, or nicotine. If the person has no heart ailment, treatment is rarely done.

## *Other Arrhythmias*

There are other arrhythmias under some of these categories. Some could be congenital while others are caused by other factors like the presence of implants and other medical conditions. Admittedly, some of these arrhythmias may have the same ECG tracings, which makes it possible to overlook any difference. With practice though, one will become an expert in interpreting ECG's.

# Chapter 6:
# Tips For a Healthy Heart: No to Arrhythmias

It is possible to prevent arrhythmias. Wouldn't it be nice to have normal ECG readings after every test? It is possible when you have a healthy heart. Here are 12 simple tips to follow:

1. Healthy diet. Most of the time, people know what is and what is not good for them. It is not a lack of knowledge that leads to obesity or heart ailments, but the lack of discipline and compliance to the recommended diet. You can choose from many dietary programs. Pick one that is suitable for your schedule, personality and target weight. Maintaining an ideal weight is one way of keeping your heart healthy. In addition, avoiding foods that can harm your heart (such as fatty, salty, processed foods) can result in a happy and healthy heart.

2. Exercise and activity. Time and time again, the importance of exercise has been emphasized. Still, many people follow a sedentary lifestyle. Exercise is not only good for the heart, but for your overall health - mental, psychological, social and even spiritual health.

3. Smoking Cessation. Nicotine is the main culprit for the millions of preventable deaths in the world today. A study has revealed that for every cigarette that is smoked, an average of seven minutes is deducted from one's life.

4. Stress Management. Almost 85% of all diseases can be traced back to stress as the causative factor. There are many relaxation techniques and stress management programs that one can take to eliminate unnecessary anxieties in one's life. One suggestion is to take a hobby

that you really like and try to spend one hour a day just enjoying your hobby.

5. Cessation of Alcohol Consumption. Alcohol is not only fattening, but it is so harmful to the liver. The heart suffers from an excessive intake of alcohol due to obesity, hypertension, stroke and other medical problems.

6. Have Regular Check Ups. Visit your primary health care provider on a regular basis, especially if you have existing medical conditions. The heart is treacherous thing. You may feel fine today and be really sick tomorrow. Do not wait for the condition to worsen. Prevention is really better than an ounce of cure, as the saying goes.

7. Sleep and Rest. One of the challenges facing today's generation is the lack of adequate rest and sleep. There are always things to do. 24 hours is not enough, but the heart needs to rest, too. Not giving it enough time to recharge and recuperate could wear your heart out earlier.

8. Laugh out loud. Laughter is indeed a great medicine for the heart. Studies prove that even if you laugh without any reason, you are giving your heart a boost. However, when you laugh heartily, your heart benefits a lot.

9. Improve your Sex Life. Having more time to enjoy your partner in bed is good for your heart and for your marriage or relationship. According to studies, sexual intercourse is equivalent to a 30-minute heavy workout.

10. Eat Chocolates. Don't feel guilty either! However, the recommended chocolates are the dark ones. Why chocolates? They contain flavonoids that could keep heart diseases at bay. In addition, they are also known to make one feel good emotionally. This means lesser stress and anxieties.

11. Own a pet. Another treat for the heart is having a pet to love. There is a lower incidence of deaths from heart diseases when the person owns a pet, as revealed by studies of the National Health Institute.

12. Go out and have fun. Being with other people and simply enjoying your life can improve the condition of the heart. Volunteer to a worthy cause or just spend more quality time with friends and families. These simple activities can make your heart healthier and your life happier.

Take care of your heart and it will take care of you. The bottom line of ECG interpretation is to understand your heart and aspire to keep it in good shape at all times.

# Conclusion

Thank you again for downloading this book!

I hope this book was able to help you learn more about ECG interpretation!

The next step is to put this information to use, and begin interpreting the different rhythms of your heart!

Finally, if you enjoyed this book, please take the time to share your thoughts and post a review on Amazon. It'd be greatly appreciated!

Thank you and good luck!

www.ingramcontent.com/pod-product-compliance
Lightning Source LLC
Chambersburg PA
CBHW072200060526
44654CB00046B/1368